TYPE 1 DIABETES KID-FRIENDLY VEGETARIAN RECIPES

Delicious and Fun Plant-Based Meals That Kids Love! Expertly Crafted to Support Healthy Blood Sugar Levels for Children

By Mia Bennett

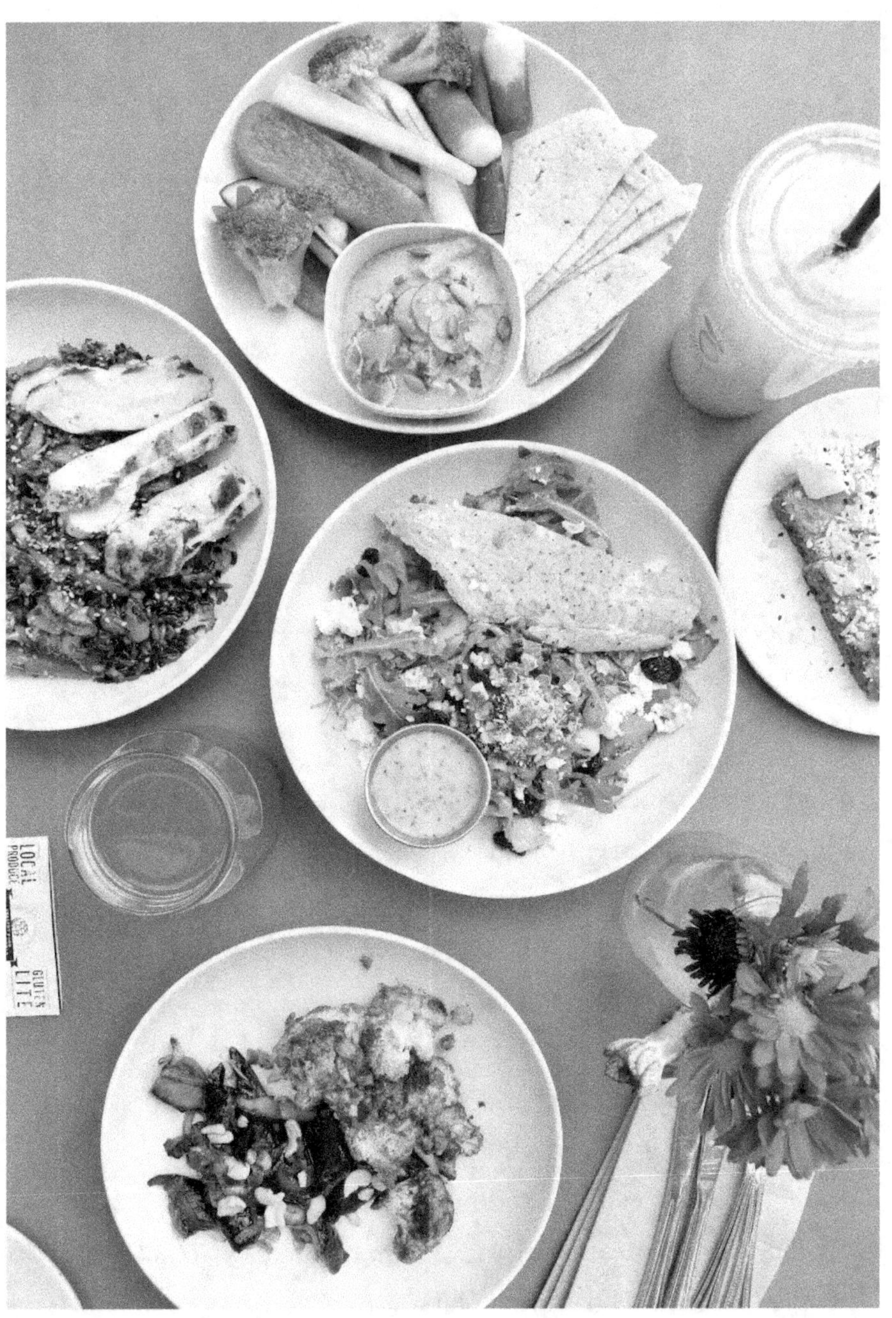

TABLE OF CONTENTS

Chapter 3: Lunch Recipes 39

Chapter 4: Dinner Recipes 57

Chapter 5: Snacks and Appetizers 76

INTRODUCTION

I magine a world where your child's favorite foods suddenly become a puzzle to solve. This is the reality for families living with Type 1 Diabetes (T1D) in children. The body stops producing insulin, a hormone crucial for converting food into energy, leaving parents grappling with questions about meals and managing blood sugar levels.

Here's a roadmap to navigate this journey, focusing on the power of a balanced vegetarian diet:

Understanding Type 1 Diabetes in Children:

- **The Body's Balancing Act:** Unlike Type 2 Diabetes, T1D isn't caused by lifestyle choices. The immune system mistakenly attacks insulin-producing cells in the pancreas.
- **Fueling the Engine:** Food breaks down into glucose (sugar) absorbed by cells with the help of insulin. Without insulin, glucose builds up in the bloodstream, leading to health complications if not managed.

Why a Balanced Vegetarian Diet is Important:

- **Fiber Powerhouse:** Plant-based diets are naturally high in fiber, which slows down glucose absorption, promoting steadier blood sugar levels.

- **Vitamin and Mineral Bounty**: A vegetarian plate brimming with colorful vegetables, fruits, and whole grains provides essential vitamins and minerals for overall growth and development.

- **Healthy Weight Management:** Vegetarian diets tend to be lower in saturated fat and cholesterol, promoting a healthy weight, which can further improve blood sugar control.

Key Nutrients for Diabetic Children:

- **Protein Power:** Include lean protein sources like beans, lentils, tofu, and nuts in every meal. Protein helps with satiety and slows down digestion, preventing blood sugar spikes.

- **Healthy Fats:** Don't shy away from healthy fats like avocados, nuts, and seeds. These fats keep your child feeling full and provide essential fatty acids for growth.

- **Carbohydrate Choices:** Focus on complex carbohydrates found in whole grains, legumes, and non-starchy vegetables.

These provide sustained energy without causing rapid blood sugar spikes.

Tips for Meal Planning and Preparation:

- **Teamwork Makes the Dream Work:** Involve your child in meal planning. Let them choose recipes, pick out vegetables at the grocery store, and help with age-appropriate tasks in the kitchen. This fosters a sense of ownership and builds healthy habits.

- **Planning is Key:** Prepare a weekly meal plan considering your child's activities and insulin needs. Prepping snacks and chopping vegetables in advance saves time and prevents last-minute unhealthy choices.

- **Portion Control is Essential:** Work with a registered dietitian to create a personalized meal plan with appropriate portion sizes for your child's age and activity level.

- **Variety is the Spice of Life:** Explore the vibrant world of vegetarian cuisine! Experiment with different ethnic flavors, textures, and colors to keep mealtimes exciting and ensure a well-rounded intake of nutrients.

Remember: You're not alone on this journey. Connect with support groups, consult a registered dietitian specializing in pediatric diabetes, and celebrate every milestone. With a balanced vegetarian diet, careful planning, and a positive attitude, you can empower your child to thrive with T1D.

Chapter 1: 30 Day Meal Plan

Week 1

Day 1:

- Breakfast: Blueberry Oatmeal
- Lunch: Chickpea Salad Sandwich
- Dinner: Eggplant Parmesan
- Snack: Roasted Chickpeas
- Dessert: Sugar-Free Chocolate Avocado Mousse

Day 2:

- Breakfast: Veggie Scramble with Tofu
- Lunch: Spinach and Feta Stuffed Peppers
- Dinner: Stuffed Zucchini Boats
- Snack: Cucumber and Hummus Bites
- Dessert: Baked Cinnamon Apples

Day 3:

- Breakfast: Avocado Toast with Cherry Tomatoes
- Lunch: Veggie and Hummus Wrap
- Dinner: Vegetable Curry with Brown Rice
- Snack: Apple Slices with Peanut Butter
- Dessert: Chia Seed Pudding with Coconut Milk

Day 4:

- Breakfast: Spinach and Mushroom Breakfast Wrap
- Lunch: Quinoa and Black Bean Salad
- Dinner: Baked Tofu with Steamed Broccoli
- Snack: Veggie Sticks with Greek Yogurt Dip
- Dessert: Greek Yogurt with Honey and Berries

Day 5:

- Breakfast: Chia Seed Pudding with Fresh Berries
- Lunch: Lentil Soup with Carrots and Celery
- Dinner: Spaghetti Squash with Marinara Sauce
- Snack: Mini Caprese Skewers
- Dessert: Almond Flour Brownies

Day 6:

- Breakfast: Whole Wheat Pancakes with Sugar-Free Syrup
- Lunch: Tofu and Veggie Stir-Fry
- Dinner: Lentil and Vegetable Shepherd's Pie
- Snack: Edamame with Sea Salt
- Dessert: Frozen Banana Pops with Dark Chocolate

Day 7:

- Breakfast: Greek Yogurt with Nuts and Seeds
- Lunch: Roasted Vegetable Quinoa Bowl

- Dinner: Mushroom Risotto

- Snack: Guacamole with Carrot Sticks

- Dessert: Carrot and Pineapple Muffins

Week 2

Day 8:

- Breakfast: Quinoa Breakfast Bowl with Almonds

- Lunch: Caprese Salad with Basil and Balsamic

- Dinner: Stuffed Bell Peppers with Quinoa and Spinach

- Snack: Baked Zucchini Chips

- Dessert: Raspberry Sorbet

Day 9:

- Breakfast: Smoothie Bowl with Mixed Fruits

- Lunch: Greek Salad with Chickpeas

- Dinner: Thai Red Curry with Tofu

- Snack: Almond Flour Crackers with Cheese

- Dessert: Coconut Macaroons

Day 10:

- Breakfast: Zucchini and Carrot Muffins

- Lunch: Mushroom and Spinach Quesadilla

- Dinner: Cauliflower Fried Rice

- Snack: Stuffed Mini Bell Peppers
- Dessert: Mango and Lime Sorbet

Day 11:

- Breakfast: Apple Cinnamon Overnight Oats
- Lunch: Baked Sweet Potato with Black Beans and Corn
- Dinner: Vegetable Lasagna with Whole Wheat Noodles
- Snack: Cauliflower Buffalo Bites
- Dessert: Vegan Chocolate Chip Cookies

Day 12:

- Breakfast: Cottage Cheese with Pineapple and Mint
- Lunch: Pasta Primavera with Zoodles
- Dinner: Spinach and Ricotta Stuffed Shells
- Snack: Mixed Nuts and Seeds
- Dessert: Lemon Blueberry Bars

Day 13:

- Breakfast: Almond Butter and Banana Sandwich
- Lunch: Cauliflower Tacos with Lime Crema
- Dinner: Grilled Veggie Kabobs
- Snack: Tofu Nuggets with Dipping Sauce
- Dessert: Strawberry Shortcake

Day 14:

- Breakfast: Savory Lentil Pancakes
- Lunch: Asian Noodle Salad with Peanut Dressing
- Dinner: Vegan Chili with Kidney Beans
- Snack: Sweet Potato Fries with Cinnamon
- Dessert: Pomegranate and Orange Salad

Week 3

Day 15:

- Breakfast: Broccoli and Cheese Frittata
- Lunch: Grilled Portobello Mushroom Burger
- Dinner: Butternut Squash and Kale Salad
- Snack: Fruit Salad with Mint
- Dessert: Vegan Banana Bread

Day 16:

- Breakfast: Blueberry Oatmeal
- Lunch: Chickpea Salad Sandwich
- Dinner: Eggplant Parmesan
- Snack: Roasted Chickpeas
- Dessert: Sugar-Free Chocolate Avocado Mousse

Day 17:

- Breakfast: Veggie Scramble with Tofu
- Lunch: Spinach and Feta Stuffed Peppers
- Dinner: Stuffed Zucchini Boats
- Snack: Cucumber and Hummus Bites
- Dessert: Baked Cinnamon Apples

Day 18:

- Breakfast: Avocado Toast with Cherry Tomatoes
- Lunch: Veggie and Hummus Wrap
- Dinner: Vegetable Curry with Brown Rice
- Snack: Apple Slices with Peanut Butter
- Dessert: Chia Seed Pudding with Coconut Milk

Day 19:

- Breakfast: Spinach and Mushroom Breakfast Wrap
- Lunch: Quinoa and Black Bean Salad
- Dinner: Baked Tofu with Steamed Broccoli
- Snack: Veggie Sticks with Greek Yogurt Dip
- Dessert: Greek Yogurt with Honey and Berries

Day 20:

- Breakfast: Chia Seed Pudding with Fresh Berries
- Lunch: Lentil Soup with Carrots and Celery

- Dinner: Spaghetti Squash with Marinara Sauce

- Snack: Mini Caprese Skewers

- Dessert: Almond Flour Brownies

Day 21:

- Breakfast: Whole Wheat Pancakes with Sugar-Free Syrup

- Lunch: Tofu and Veggie Stir-Fry

- Dinner: Lentil and Vegetable Shepherd's Pie

- Snack: Edamame with Sea Salt

- Dessert: Frozen Banana Pops with Dark Chocolate

Week 4

Day 22:

- Breakfast: Greek Yogurt with Nuts and Seeds

- Lunch: Roasted Vegetable Quinoa Bowl

- Dinner: Mushroom Risotto

- Snack: Guacamole with Carrot Sticks

- Dessert: Carrot and Pineapple Muffins

Day 23:

- Breakfast: Quinoa Breakfast Bowl with Almonds

- Lunch: Caprese Salad with Basil and Balsamic

- Dinner: Stuffed Bell Peppers with Quinoa and Spinach

- Snack: Baked Zucchini Chips
- Dessert: Raspberry Sorbet

Day 24:

- Breakfast: Smoothie Bowl with Mixed Fruits
- Lunch: Greek Salad with Chickpeas
- Dinner: Thai Red Curry with Tofu
- Snack: Almond Flour Crackers with Cheese
- Dessert: Coconut Macaroons

Day 25:

- Breakfast: Zucchini and Carrot Muffins
- Lunch: Mushroom and Spinach Quesadilla
- Dinner: Cauliflower Fried Rice
- Snack: Stuffed Mini Bell Peppers
- Dessert: Mango and Lime Sorbet

Day 26:

- Breakfast: Apple Cinnamon Overnight Oats
- Lunch: Baked Sweet Potato with Black Beans and Corn
- Dinner: Vegetable Lasagna with Whole Wheat Noodles
- Snack: Cauliflower Buffalo Bites
- Dessert: Vegan Chocolate Chip Cookies

Day 27:

- Breakfast: Cottage Cheese with Pineapple and Mint
- Lunch: Pasta Primavera with Zoodles
- Dinner: Spinach and Ricotta Stuffed Shells
- Snack: Mixed Nuts and Seeds
- Dessert: Lemon Blueberry Bars

Day 28:

- Breakfast: Almond Butter and Banana Sandwich
- Lunch: Cauliflower Tacos with Lime Crema
- Dinner: Grilled Veggie Kabobs
- Snack: Tofu Nuggets with Dipping Sauce
- Dessert: Strawberry Shortcake

Day 29:

- Breakfast: Savory Lentil Pancakes
- Lunch: Asian Noodle Salad with Peanut Dressing
- Dinner: Vegan Chili with Kidney Beans
- Snack: Sweet Potato Fries with Cinnamon
- Dessert: Pomegranate and Orange Salad

Day 30:

- Breakfast: Broccoli and Cheese Frittata
- Lunch: Grilled Portobello Mushroom Burger

- Dinner: Butternut Squash and Kale Salad

- Snack: Fruit Salad with Mint

- Dessert: Vegan Banana Bread

Chapter 2: Breakfast Recipes

Starting your day with a healthy, balanced breakfast is especially important for children with Type 1 diabetes. These kid-friendly vegetarian breakfast recipes are designed to provide essential nutrients while keeping blood sugar levels stable. Each recipe is easy to prepare and packed with flavors that kids will love.

Blueberry Oatmeal

Ingredients:

- 1 cup rolled oats
- 2 cups water or unsweetened almond milk
- 1/2 cup fresh or frozen blueberries
- 1 tsp cinnamon
- 1 tbsp chia seeds
- 1 tsp vanilla extract
- 1 tbsp maple syrup (optional)

Instructions:

1. In a saucepan, bring water or almond milk to a boil.
2. Add oats and reduce heat to simmer.
3. Stir in blueberries, cinnamon, chia seeds, and vanilla extract.
4. Cook for 5-7 minutes, stirring occasionally until thickened.

5. Serve warm with a drizzle of maple syrup if desired.

Nutrition Information (per serving):

- Calories: 220
- Protein: 6g
- Carbohydrates: 38g
- Fat: 5g
- Fiber: 7g
- Sugar: 7g
- Portion size: 1 cup

Veggie Scramble with Tofu

Ingredients:

- 1 block firm tofu, crumbled
- 1 tbsp olive oil
- 1/2 cup diced bell peppers
- 1/2 cup diced tomatoes
- 1/2 cup spinach leaves
- 1/4 cup diced onions
- 1 tsp turmeric
- Salt and pepper to taste

Instructions:

1. Heat olive oil in a skillet over medium heat.

2. Add onions, bell peppers, and tomatoes; sauté for 3-4 minutes.

3. Add crumbled tofu and turmeric; cook for 5 minutes.

4. Stir in spinach and cook until wilted.

5. Season with salt and pepper.

Nutrition Information (per serving):

- Calories: 180
- Protein: 14g
- Carbohydrates: 8g
- Fat: 11g
- Fiber: 3g
- Sugar: 3g
- Portion size: 1 cup

Avocado Toast with Cherry Tomatoes

Ingredients:

- 1 slice whole grain bread
- 1/2 avocado, mashed
- 1/4 cup cherry tomatoes, halved
- Salt and pepper to taste

- 1 tbsp olive oil

Instructions:

1. Toast the bread.
2. Spread mashed avocado over the toast.
3. Top with cherry tomatoes.
4. Drizzle with olive oil and season with salt and pepper.

Nutrition Information (per serving):

- Calories: 250
- Protein: 4g
- Carbohydrates: 25g
- Fat: 18g
- Fiber: 7g
- Sugar: 3g
- Portion size: 1 slice

Spinach and Mushroom Breakfast Wrap

Ingredients:

- 1 whole wheat tortilla
- 1/2 cup sliced mushrooms
- 1/2 cup fresh spinach
- 1/4 cup shredded cheese (optional)

- 1 tbsp olive oil

Instructions:

1. Heat olive oil in a pan over medium heat.
2. Sauté mushrooms until tender.
3. Add spinach and cook until wilted.
4. Place the mixture on the tortilla and sprinkle with cheese.
5. Roll up the tortilla and serve warm.

Nutrition Information (per serving):

- Calories: 220
- Protein: 7g
- Carbohydrates: 22g
- Fat: 12g
- Fiber: 4g
- Sugar: 2g
- Portion size: 1 wrap

Chia Seed Pudding with Fresh Berries

Ingredients:

- 1/4 cup chia seeds
- 1 cup unsweetened almond milk
- 1 tsp vanilla extract

- 1 tbsp maple syrup (optional)
- 1/2 cup mixed fresh berries

Instructions:

1. Mix chia seeds, almond milk, vanilla extract, and maple syrup in a bowl.
2. Refrigerate for at least 4 hours or overnight.
3. Top with fresh berries before serving.

Nutrition Information (per serving):

- Calories: 190
- Protein: 5g
- Carbohydrates: 25g
- Fat: 8g
- Fiber: 10g
- Sugar: 9g
- Portion size: 1 cup

Whole Wheat Pancakes with Sugar-Free Syrup

Ingredients:

- 1 cup whole wheat flour
- 1 tbsp baking powder

- 1/2 tsp salt
- 1 cup unsweetened almond milk
- 1 egg
- 1 tbsp coconut oil, melted
- Sugar-free syrup

Instructions:

1. Mix flour, baking powder, and salt in a bowl.
2. In another bowl, whisk almond milk, egg, and melted coconut oil.
3. Combine wet and dry ingredients; stir until smooth.
4. Cook pancakes on a griddle over medium heat until bubbles form.
5. Serve with sugar-free syrup.

Nutrition Information (per serving):

- Calories: 160
- Protein: 6g
- Carbohydrates: 25g
- Fat: 4g
- Fiber: 4g
- Sugar: 0g
- Portion size: 2 pancakes

Greek Yogurt with Nuts and Seeds

Ingredients:

- 1 cup plain Greek yogurt
- 2 tbsp mixed nuts (almonds, walnuts, pistachios)
- 1 tbsp chia seeds
- 1 tbsp flaxseeds
- 1 tsp honey (optional)

Instructions:

1. Scoop Greek yogurt into a bowl.
2. Top with mixed nuts, chia seeds, and flaxseeds.
3. Drizzle with honey if desired.

Nutrition Information (per serving):

- Calories: 200
- Protein: 15g
- Carbohydrates: 15g
- Fat: 10g
- Fiber: 5g
- Sugar: 8g
- Portion size: 1 cup

Quinoa Breakfast Bowl with Almonds

Ingredients:

- 1/2 cup cooked quinoa
- 1/4 cup almond milk
- 1 tbsp almond butter
- 1 tbsp sliced almonds
- 1/2 apple, chopped
- 1 tsp cinnamon

Instructions:

1. Warm cooked quinoa in a saucepan with almond milk.
2. Stir in almond butter and cinnamon.
3. Top with sliced almonds and chopped apple.

Nutrition Information (per serving):

- Calories: 250
- Protein: 7g
- Carbohydrates: 30g
- Fat: 10g
- Fiber: 6g
- Sugar: 8g
- Portion size: 1 bowl

Smoothie Bowl with Mixed Fruits

Ingredients:

- 1 banana
- 1/2 cup frozen berries
- 1/2 cup unsweetened almond milk
- 1 tbsp chia seeds
- 1/4 cup granola
- 1/4 cup fresh mixed fruits

Instructions:

1. Blend banana, frozen berries, almond milk, and chia seeds until smooth.
2. Pour into a bowl and top with granola and fresh fruits.

Nutrition Information (per serving):

- Calories: 300
- Protein: 5g
- Carbohydrates: 60g
- Fat: 8g
- Fiber: 10g
- Sugar: 25g
- Portion size: 1 bowl

Zucchini and Carrot Muffins

Ingredients:

- 1 cup grated zucchini
- 1 cup grated carrots
- 1 cup whole wheat flour
- 1 tsp baking powder
- 1/2 tsp baking soda
- 1/2 tsp cinnamon
- 1/4 cup coconut oil, melted
- 1/2 cup unsweetened applesauce
- 1 egg

Instructions:

1. Preheat oven to 350°F (175°C).
2. Mix flour, baking powder, baking soda, and cinnamon in a bowl.
3. In another bowl, combine coconut oil, applesauce, and egg.
4. Stir in grated zucchini and carrots.
5. Mix wet and dry ingredients until just combined.
6. Pour batter into muffin cups and bake for 20-25 minutes.

Nutrition Information (per serving):

- Calories: 150
- Protein: 3g

- Carbohydrates: 18g

- Fat: 7g

- Fiber: 3g

- Sugar: 7g

- Portion size: 1 muffin

Apple Cinnamon Overnight Oats

Ingredients:

- 1/2 cup rolled oats

- 1/2 cup unsweetened almond milk

- 1/2 apple, chopped

- 1 tsp cinnamon

- 1 tbsp chia seeds

- 1 tsp maple syrup (optional)

Instructions:

1. Combine all ingredients in a jar.

2. Stir well and refrigerate overnight.

3. Serve chilled or warm up slightly before eating.

Nutrition Information (per serving):

- Calories: 220

- Protein: 6g

- Carbohydrates: 38g

- Fat: 5g

- Fiber: 7g

- Sugar: 9g

- Portion size: 1 cup

Cottage Cheese with Pineapple and Mint

Ingredients:

- 1 cup cottage cheese

- 1/2 cup pineapple chunks

- 1 tbsp fresh mint, chopped

Instructions:

1. Mix cottage cheese and pineapple chunks in a bowl.

2. Top with chopped mint.

Nutrition Information (per serving):

- Calories: 180

- Protein: 14g

- Carbohydrates: 12g

- Fat: 6g

- Fiber: 1g

- Sugar: 9g

- Portion size: 1 cup

Almond Butter and Banana Sandwich

Ingredients:

- 2 slices whole grain bread
- 2 tbsp almond butter
- 1 banana, sliced

Instructions:

1. Spread almond butter on one slice of bread.
2. Layer banana slices on top.
3. Cover with the second slice of bread.

Nutrition Information (per serving):

- Calories: 300
- Protein: 9g
- Carbohydrates: 42g
- Fat: 12g
- Fiber: 7g
- Sugar: 10g
- Portion size: 1 sandwich

Savory Lentil Pancakes

Ingredients:

- 1 cup lentil flour
- 1/2 cup water
- 1/4 cup chopped spinach
- 1/4 cup grated carrots
- Salt and pepper to taste
- 1 tbsp olive oil

Instructions:

1. Mix lentil flour and water to form a batter.
2. Stir in chopped spinach, grated carrots, salt, and pepper.
3. Heat olive oil in a pan and pour batter to form pancakes.
4. Cook until golden on both sides.

Nutrition Information (per serving):

- Calories: 160
- Protein: 8g
- Carbohydrates: 20g
- Fat: 5g
- Fiber: 5g
- Sugar: 2g
- Portion size: 2 pancakes

Broccoli and Cheese Frittata

Ingredients:

- 1 cup broccoli florets, chopped
- 4 eggs
- 1/4 cup milk
- 1/2 cup shredded cheese
- Salt and pepper to taste

Instructions:

1. Preheat oven to 350°F (175°C).
2. Steam broccoli until tender.
3. Beat eggs with milk, salt, and pepper.
4. Stir in steamed broccoli and cheese.
5. Pour mixture into a greased baking dish and bake for 20-25 minutes.

Nutrition Information (per serving):

- Calories: 250
- Protein: 16g
- Carbohydrates: 6g
- Fat: 18g
- Fiber: 2g
- Sugar: 2g
- Portion size: 1 slice

Chapter 3: Lunch Recipes

Creating nutritious and delicious lunches for children with Type 1 Diabetes can be a challenge, but it's certainly possible with the right recipes. These vegetarian lunch recipes are not only kid-friendly but also balanced to help manage blood sugar levels. Each recipe is designed to be easy to prepare and enjoyable for the whole family.

Chickpea Salad Sandwich

Ingredients:

- 1 can chickpeas, drained and mashed
- 2 tbsp Greek yogurt
- 1 tbsp Dijon mustard
- 1 celery stalk, chopped
- 1 small carrot, grated
- 1 tbsp chopped parsley
- Salt and pepper to taste
- Whole grain bread

Instructions:

1. In a bowl, combine mashed chickpeas, Greek yogurt, Dijon mustard, celery, carrot, and parsley.
2. Season with salt and pepper.

3. Spread mixture on whole grain bread and assemble sandwich.

Nutrition Information (per sandwich):
- Calories: 320
- Protein: 14g
- Carbohydrates: 52g
- Fat: 6g
- Fiber: 12g
- Sugar: 5g
- Portion Size: 1 sandwich

Spinach and Feta Stuffed Peppers

Ingredients:
- 4 bell peppers, halved and seeded
- 1 cup cooked quinoa
- 1 cup fresh spinach, chopped
- 1/2 cup feta cheese, crumbled
- 1 small onion, diced
- 1 clove garlic, minced
- 1 tbsp olive oil
- Salt and pepper to taste

Instructions:

1. Preheat oven to 375°F (190°C).
2. Sauté onion and garlic in olive oil until soft.
3. Combine quinoa, spinach, feta, and sautéed onion mixture in a bowl.
4. Stuff peppers with mixture and place in baking dish.
5. Bake for 20-25 minutes until peppers are tender.

Nutrition Information (per serving):

- Calories: 210
- Protein: 7g
- Carbohydrates: 27g
- Fat: 9g
- Fiber: 5g
- Sugar: 6g
- Portion Size: 2 stuffed pepper halves

Veggie and Hummus Wrap

Ingredients:

- 1 whole wheat tortilla
- 3 tbsp hummus
- 1/4 cup shredded carrots
- 1/4 cup sliced cucumber

- 1/4 cup bell pepper strips
- Handful of spinach leaves

Instructions:

1. Spread hummus over tortilla.
2. Layer with carrots, cucumber, bell pepper, and spinach.
3. Roll up the tortilla tightly and slice in half.

Nutrition Information (per wrap):

- Calories: 220
- Protein: 6g
- Carbohydrates: 34g
- Fat: 8g
- Fiber: 7g
- Sugar: 4g
- Portion Size: 1 wrap

Quinoa and Black Bean Salad

Ingredients:

- 1 cup cooked quinoa
- 1 can black beans, drained and rinsed
- 1 cup cherry tomatoes, halved
- 1/4 cup chopped red onion

- 1/4 cup chopped cilantro
- Juice of 1 lime
- 2 tbsp olive oil
- Salt and pepper to taste

Instructions:

1. In a large bowl, combine quinoa, black beans, tomatoes, red onion, and cilantro.
2. Whisk together lime juice, olive oil, salt, and pepper.
3. Pour dressing over salad and toss to combine.

Nutrition Information (per serving):

- Calories: 250
- Protein: 9g
- Carbohydrates: 36g
- Fat: 8g
- Fiber: 10g
- Sugar: 2g
- Portion Size: 1 cup

Lentil Soup with Carrots and Celery

Ingredients:

- 1 cup dried lentils, rinsed

- 1 large carrot, chopped
- 2 celery stalks, chopped
- 1 small onion, diced
- 2 cloves garlic, minced
- 4 cups vegetable broth
- 1 bay leaf
- 1 tbsp olive oil
- Salt and pepper to taste

Instructions:

1. Sauté onion, garlic, carrot, and celery in olive oil until softened.
2. Add lentils, vegetable broth, and bay leaf.
3. Simmer for 30-40 minutes until lentils are tender.
4. Season with salt and pepper.

Nutrition Information (per serving):

- Calories: 180
- Protein: 11g
- Carbohydrates: 31g
- Fat: 3g
- Fiber: 14g
- Sugar: 4g
- Portion Size: 1 cup

Tofu and Veggie Stir-Fry

Ingredients:

- 1 block firm tofu, cubed
- 2 cups mixed vegetables (bell peppers, broccoli, snap peas)
- 2 tbsp soy sauce
- 1 tbsp sesame oil
- 1 clove garlic, minced
- 1 tsp grated ginger
- 1 tbsp sesame seeds

Instructions:

1. Sauté tofu in sesame oil until golden brown.
2. Add garlic and ginger, cook for 1 minute.
3. Add mixed vegetables and soy sauce, stir-fry until vegetables are tender.
4. Sprinkle with sesame seeds before serving.

Nutrition Information (per serving):

- Calories: 220
- Protein: 15g
- Carbohydrates: 12g
- Fat: 14g
- Fiber: 4g
- Sugar: 3g

- Portion Size: 1 cup

Roasted Vegetable Quinoa Bowl

Ingredients:

- 1 cup cooked quinoa
- 1 cup assorted roasted vegetables (zucchini, bell peppers, carrots)
- 1 tbsp olive oil
- 1 tsp balsamic vinegar
- Salt and pepper to taste
- Fresh parsley for garnish

Instructions:

1. Toss vegetables with olive oil, salt, and pepper, then roast at 400°F (200°C) for 20 minutes.
2. Combine cooked quinoa and roasted vegetables.
3. Drizzle with balsamic vinegar and garnish with parsley.

Nutrition Information (per serving):

- Calories: 230
- Protein: 6g
- Carbohydrates: 35g
- Fat: 8g

- Fiber: 6g
- Sugar: 5g
- Portion Size: 1 bowl

Caprese Salad with Basil and Balsamic

Ingredients:

- 2 cups cherry tomatoes, halved
- 1 cup fresh mozzarella balls
- 1/4 cup fresh basil leaves
- 1 tbsp balsamic vinegar
- 1 tbsp olive oil
- Salt and pepper to taste

Instructions:

1. Combine tomatoes, mozzarella, and basil in a bowl.
2. Drizzle with balsamic vinegar and olive oil.
3. Season with salt and pepper.

Nutrition Information (per serving):

- Calories: 180
- Protein: 8g
- Carbohydrates: 10g
- Fat: 13g

- Fiber: 2g

- Sugar: 6g

- Portion Size: 1 cup

Greek Salad with Chickpeas

Ingredients:

- 1 can chickpeas, drained and rinsed

- 1 cucumber, diced

- 1 cup cherry tomatoes, halved

- 1/4 cup red onion, sliced

- 1/4 cup kalamata olives, pitted

- 1/4 cup feta cheese, crumbled

- 1 tbsp olive oil

- Juice of 1 lemon

- Salt and pepper to taste

Instructions:

1. Combine chickpeas, cucumber, tomatoes, onion, olives, and feta in a bowl.

2. Drizzle with olive oil and lemon juice.

3. Season with salt and pepper.

Nutrition Information (per serving):

- Calories: 220
- Protein: 8g
- Carbohydrates: 28g
- Fat: 10g
- Fiber: 8g
- Sugar: 6g
- Portion Size: 1 cup

Mushroom and Spinach Quesadilla

Ingredients:

- 1 whole wheat tortilla
- 1/2 cup sliced mushrooms
- 1 cup fresh spinach
- 1/4 cup shredded mozzarella cheese
- 1 tsp olive oil

Instructions:

1. Sauté mushrooms in olive oil until soft.
2. Add spinach and cook until wilted.
3. Place tortilla in a pan, add mushroom-spinach mixture and cheese.
4. Fold tortilla and cook until cheese is melted.

Nutrition Information (per serving):

- Calories: 210
- Protein: 9g
- Carbohydrates: 26g
- Fat: 9g
- Fiber: 4g
- Sugar: 2g
- Portion Size: 1 quesadilla

Baked Sweet Potato with Black Beans and Corn

Ingredients:

- 2 medium sweet potatoes
- 1 cup black beans, drained and rinsed
- 1 cup corn kernels
- 1/4 cup salsa
- 1 tbsp chopped cilantro

Instructions:

1. Bake sweet potatoes at 400°F (200°C) for 45 minutes or until tender.
2. Cut sweet potatoes open and fill with black beans, corn, and salsa.

3. Sprinkle with cilantro before serving.

Nutrition Information (per serving):

- Calories: 250
- Protein: 7g
- Carbohydrates: 52g
- Fat: 2g
- Fiber: 10g
- Sugar: 12g
- Portion Size: 1 stuffed sweet potato

Pasta Primavera with Zoodles

Ingredients:

- 2 cups zucchini noodles
- 1 cup cherry tomatoes, halved
- 1/2 cup bell pepper strips
- 1/2 cup broccoli florets
- 2 tbsp olive oil
- 2 cloves garlic, minced
- Salt and pepper to taste
- Grated Parmesan for garnish

Instructions:

1. Sauté garlic in olive oil until fragrant.

2. Add vegetables and cook until tender.

3. Toss with zucchini noodles and season with salt and pepper.

4. Sprinkle with Parmesan before serving.

Nutrition Information (per serving):

- Calories: 180

- Protein: 4g

- Carbohydrates: 18g

- Fat: 12g

- Fiber: 5g

- Sugar: 7g

- Portion Size: 1 cup

Cauliflower Tacos with Lime Crema

Ingredients:

- 2 cups cauliflower florets

- 1 tbsp olive oil

- 1 tsp chili powder

- 1/2 tsp cumin

- Salt to taste

- 4 small corn tortillas

- 1/2 cup shredded cabbage
- 1/4 cup Greek yogurt
- Juice of 1 lime

Instructions:

1. Toss cauliflower with olive oil, chili powder, cumin, and salt.
2. Roast at 400°F (200°C) for 20 minutes.
3. Combine Greek yogurt and lime juice to make crema.
4. Assemble tacos with cauliflower, cabbage, and lime crema.

Nutrition Information (per serving):

- Calories: 220
- Protein: 6g
- Carbohydrates: 28g
- Fat: 10g
- Fiber: 5g
- Sugar: 4g
- Portion Size: 2 tacos

Asian Noodle Salad with Peanut Dressing

Ingredients:

- 4 oz rice noodles
- 1 cup shredded carrots
- 1 cup sliced bell peppers
- 1/2 cup chopped green onions
- 1/4 cup chopped cilantro
- 1/4 cup peanut butter
- 2 tbsp soy sauce
- 1 tbsp rice vinegar
- 1 tsp sesame oil

Instructions:

1. Cook rice noodles according to package instructions.
2. In a bowl, combine peanut butter, soy sauce, rice vinegar, and sesame oil to make dressing.
3. Toss noodles with vegetables and dressing.
4. Garnish with cilantro.

Nutrition Information (per serving):

- Calories: 310
- Protein: 8g
- Carbohydrates: 42g

- Fat: 14g
- Fiber: 4g
- Sugar: 6g
- Portion Size: 1 cup

Grilled Portobello Mushroom Burger

Ingredients:

- 4 large Portobello mushrooms, stems removed
- 2 tbsp olive oil
- 1 tbsp balsamic vinegar
- 1 tsp garlic powder
- Salt and pepper to taste
- Whole grain burger buns
- Lettuce, tomato, and onion slices

Instructions:

1. Marinate mushrooms in olive oil, balsamic vinegar, garlic powder, salt, and pepper for 15 minutes.
2. Grill mushrooms for 5-7 minutes on each side.
3. Assemble burgers with buns, grilled mushrooms, lettuce, tomato, and onion.

Nutrition Information (per serving):

- Calories: 250
- Protein: 7g
- Carbohydrates: 35g
- Fat: 10g
- Fiber: 5g
- Sugar: 7g
- Portion Size: 1 burger

Chapter 4: Dinner Recipes

In this chapter, you'll find a variety of delicious and nutritious vegetarian dinner recipes that are specifically designed for children with Type 1 Diabetes. Each recipe balances essential nutrients while being both kid-friendly and flavorful. These dishes incorporate a range of vegetables, proteins, and whole grains to ensure your child receives a well-rounded diet.

Eggplant Parmesan

Ingredients:

- 2 large eggplants, sliced into rounds
- 2 cups marinara sauce
- 1 cup shredded mozzarella cheese
- 1 cup grated Parmesan cheese
- 1 cup whole wheat breadcrumbs
- 2 eggs, beaten
- 2 tbsp olive oil
- Salt and pepper to taste

Instructions:

1. Preheat oven to 375°F (190°C).

2. Dip eggplant slices in beaten eggs, then coat with breadcrumbs.

3. Arrange on a baking sheet, drizzle with olive oil, and bake for 20 minutes, flipping halfway.

4. Spread a thin layer of marinara sauce in a baking dish, layer with eggplant slices, more sauce, and cheeses.

5. Repeat layers, finishing with cheese on top.

6. Bake for 25-30 minutes until bubbly and golden.

Nutrition Information:

- Calories: 280
- Protein: 12g
- Carbohydrates: 32g
- Fat: 12g
- Fiber: 7g
- Sugar: 10g
- Portion Size: 1 slice

Stuffed Zucchini Boats

Ingredients:

- 4 large zucchinis, halved lengthwise
- 1 cup cooked quinoa
- 1 cup diced tomatoes

- 1/2 cup chopped spinach
- 1/2 cup crumbled feta cheese
- 2 cloves garlic, minced
- Salt and pepper to taste

Instructions:

1. Preheat oven to 375°F (190°C).
2. Scoop out the zucchini centers to create boats.
3. In a bowl, mix quinoa, tomatoes, spinach, garlic, salt, and pepper.
4. Fill zucchini boats with the mixture and top with feta cheese.
5. Place on a baking sheet and bake for 25-30 minutes until zucchini is tender.

Nutrition Information:

- Calories: 210
- Protein: 8g
- Carbohydrates: 28g
- Fat: 8g
- Fiber: 5g
- Sugar: 7g
- Portion Size: 1 zucchini half

Vegetable Curry with Brown Rice

Ingredients:

- 1 cup brown rice
- 2 tbsp olive oil
- 1 onion, diced
- 2 cloves garlic, minced
- 1 tbsp curry powder
- 1 cup diced carrots
- 1 cup diced potatoes
- 1 cup cauliflower florets
- 1 can coconut milk
- Salt and pepper to taste

Instructions:

1. Cook brown rice according to package instructions.
2. In a large pot, heat olive oil and sauté onions and garlic until soft.
3. Add curry powder and stir for 1 minute.
4. Add carrots, potatoes, and cauliflower; cook for 5 minutes.
5. Pour in coconut milk, season with salt and pepper, and simmer for 20 minutes until vegetables are tender.
6. Serve over brown rice.

Nutrition Information:

- Calories: 350
- Protein: 7g
- Carbohydrates: 55g
- Fat: 13g
- Fiber: 7g
- Sugar: 5g
- Portion Size: 1 cup

Baked Tofu with Steamed Broccoli

Ingredients:

- 1 block firm tofu, pressed and cubed
- 2 tbsp soy sauce
- 1 tbsp olive oil
- 1 tbsp maple syrup
- 1 head broccoli, cut into florets
- Salt and pepper to taste

Instructions:

1. Preheat oven to 400°F (200°C).
2. Toss tofu cubes with soy sauce, olive oil, and maple syrup.
3. Spread on a baking sheet and bake for 25-30 minutes until golden.

4. Steam broccoli until tender.

5. Serve baked tofu with steamed broccoli.

Nutrition Information:

- Calories: 250
- Protein: 15g
- Carbohydrates: 15g
- Fat: 14g
- Fiber: 5g
- Sugar: 5g
- Portion Size: 1 cup

Spaghetti Squash with Marinara Sauce

Ingredients:

- 1 large spaghetti squash
- 2 cups marinara sauce
- 1/2 cup grated Parmesan cheese
- 2 tbsp olive oil
- Salt and pepper to taste

Instructions:

1. Preheat oven to 375°F (190°C).

2. Cut spaghetti squash in half, remove seeds, and drizzle with olive oil.

3. Place cut-side down on a baking sheet and bake for 40 minutes.

4. Scrape squash with a fork to create spaghetti-like strands.

5. Heat marinara sauce in a pot.

6. Serve spaghetti squash topped with marinara sauce and Parmesan cheese.

Nutrition Information:

- Calories: 200
- Protein: 5g
- Carbohydrates: 30g
- Fat: 8g
- Fiber: 5g
- Sugar: 10g
- Portion Size: 1 cup

Lentil and Vegetable Shepherd's Pie

Ingredients:

- 1 cup green lentils
- 2 cups vegetable broth
- 1 onion, diced

- 2 cloves garlic, minced
- 1 cup diced carrots
- 1 cup peas
- 4 cups mashed potatoes
- Salt and pepper to taste

Instructions:

1. Preheat oven to 375°F (190°C).
2. Cook lentils in vegetable broth until tender.
3. Sauté onions and garlic in a pan until soft, add carrots and peas, and cook until tender.
4. Mix cooked lentils and vegetables, season with salt and pepper.
5. Spread mixture in a baking dish, top with mashed potatoes.
6. Bake for 25 minutes until golden on top.

Nutrition Information:

- Calories: 300
- Protein: 12g
- Carbohydrates: 55g
- Fat: 3g
- Fiber: 10g
- Sugar: 5g
- Portion Size: 1 cup

Mushroom Risotto

Ingredients:

- 1 cup Arborio rice
- 4 cups vegetable broth
- 1 onion, diced
- 2 cloves garlic, minced
- 2 cups sliced mushrooms
- 1/2 cup grated Parmesan cheese
- 2 tbsp olive oil
- Salt and pepper to taste

Instructions:

1. Heat olive oil in a pot, sauté onions and garlic until soft.
2. Add mushrooms and cook until tender.
3. Stir in Arborio rice and cook for 2 minutes.
4. Gradually add vegetable broth, stirring constantly until absorbed.
5. Continue until rice is creamy and tender.
6. Stir in Parmesan cheese, season with salt and pepper.

Nutrition Information:

- Calories: 280
- Protein: 8g
- Carbohydrates: 45g

- Fat: 8g
- Fiber: 3g
- Sugar: 3g
- Portion Size: 1 cup

Stuffed Bell Peppers with Quinoa and Spinach

Ingredients:

- 4 bell peppers, tops removed and seeded
- 1 cup cooked quinoa
- 1 cup chopped spinach
- 1/2 cup diced tomatoes
- 1/2 cup shredded mozzarella cheese
- 2 cloves garlic, minced
- Salt and pepper to taste

Instructions:

1. Preheat oven to 375°F (190°C).
2. In a bowl, mix quinoa, spinach, tomatoes, garlic, salt, and pepper.
3. Fill bell peppers with the mixture and top with mozzarella cheese.
4. Place peppers in a baking dish and bake for 30 minutes.

Nutrition Information:

- Calories: 250
- Protein: 10g
- Carbohydrates: 35g
- Fat: 8g
- Fiber: 7g
- Sugar: 8g
- Portion Size: 1 pepper

Thai Red Curry with Tofu

Ingredients:

- 1 block firm tofu, cubed
- 2 tbsp red curry paste
- 1 can coconut milk
- 1 cup diced carrots
- 1 cup bell pepper strips
- 1 cup snap peas
- 2 tbsp olive oil
- Salt and pepper to taste

Instructions:

1. Heat olive oil in a pot, add red curry paste and stir for 1 minute.

2. Add coconut milk and bring to a simmer.

3. Add tofu, carrots, bell peppers, and snap peas.

4. Cook until vegetables are tender and sauce thickens.

5. Season with salt and pepper.

Nutrition Information:

- Calories: 320

- Protein: 12g

- Carbohydrates: 20g

- Fat: 24g

- Fiber: 5g

- Sugar: 7g

- Portion Size: 1 cup

Cauliflower Fried Rice

Ingredients:

- 1 head cauliflower, grated

- 2 eggs, beaten

- 1 cup peas and carrots mix

- 1 onion, diced

- 2 cloves garlic, minced

- 2 tbsp soy sauce

- 2 tbsp olive oil

- Salt and pepper to taste

Instructions:

1. Heat olive oil in a pan, sauté onions and garlic until soft.

2. Add peas and carrots, cook until tender.

3. Stir in grated cauliflower and cook for 5 minutes.

4. Push mixture to one side, scramble eggs on the other side.

5. Combine everything, add soy sauce, salt, and pepper.

Nutrition Information:

- Calories: 200

- Protein: 8g

- Carbohydrates: 18g

- Fat: 10g

- Fiber: 5g

- Sugar: 5g

- Portion Size: 1 cup

Vegetable Lasagna with Whole Wheat Noodles

Ingredients:

- 9 whole wheat lasagna noodles

- 2 cups ricotta cheese

- 2 cups shredded mozzarella cheese
- 1 cup grated Parmesan cheese
- 2 cups marinara sauce
- 1 cup spinach, chopped
- 1 cup mushrooms, sliced
- 1 zucchini, sliced
- Salt and pepper to taste

Instructions:

1. Preheat oven to 375°F (190°C).
2. Cook lasagna noodles according to package instructions.
3. Layer noodles, ricotta, spinach, mushrooms, zucchini, marinara, and cheeses in a baking dish.
4. Repeat layers, ending with cheese on top.
5. Bake for 35-40 minutes until bubbly and golden.

Nutrition Information:

- Calories: 350
- Protein: 18g
- Carbohydrates: 45g
- Fat: 12g
- Fiber: 7g
- Sugar: 10g
- Portion Size: 1 slice

Spinach and Ricotta Stuffed Shells

Ingredients:

- 20 large pasta shells
- 1 cup ricotta cheese
- 1 cup chopped spinach
- 1 cup shredded mozzarella cheese
- 1/2 cup grated Parmesan cheese
- 2 cups marinara sauce
- 1 egg, beaten
- Salt and pepper to taste

Instructions:

1. Preheat oven to 375°F (190°C).
2. Cook pasta shells according to package instructions.
3. Mix ricotta, spinach, egg, salt, and pepper in a bowl.
4. Stuff each shell with the mixture and place in a baking dish.
5. Pour marinara sauce over shells and top with mozzarella and Parmesan.
6. Bake for 25-30 minutes.

Nutrition Information:

- Calories: 300
- Protein: 15g
- Carbohydrates: 40g

- Fat: 10g
- Fiber: 5g
- Sugar: 8g
- Portion Size: 4 shells

Grilled Veggie Kabobs

Ingredients:

- 1 zucchini, sliced
- 1 bell pepper, chopped
- 1 red onion, chopped
- 1 cup cherry tomatoes
- 1/4 cup olive oil
- 2 tbsp balsamic vinegar
- Salt and pepper to taste

Instructions:

1. Preheat grill to medium-high heat.
2. Thread zucchini, bell pepper, onion, and tomatoes onto skewers.
3. Mix olive oil, balsamic vinegar, salt, and pepper; brush over skewers.
4. Grill for 10-12 minutes, turning occasionally.

Nutrition Information:

- Calories: 150
- Protein: 2g
- Carbohydrates: 10g
- Fat: 12g
- Fiber: 3g
- Sugar: 6g
- Portion Size: 2 skewers

Vegan Chili with Kidney Beans

Ingredients:

- 1 can kidney beans, drained and rinsed
- 1 can black beans, drained and rinsed
- 1 can diced tomatoes
- 1 onion, diced
- 2 cloves garlic, minced
- 1 cup corn kernels
- 2 tbsp chili powder
- 1 tbsp olive oil
- Salt and pepper to taste

Instructions:

1. Heat olive oil in a pot, sauté onions and garlic until soft.

2. Add beans, tomatoes, corn, chili powder, salt, and pepper.

3. Simmer for 20-25 minutes, stirring occasionally.

Nutrition Information:

- Calories: 220
- Protein: 10g
- Carbohydrates: 40g
- Fat: 4g
- Fiber: 10g
- Sugar: 6g
- Portion Size: 1 cup

Butternut Squash and Kale Salad

Ingredients:

- 1 small butternut squash, peeled and cubed
- 2 cups chopped kale
- 1/4 cup olive oil
- 2 tbsp balsamic vinegar
- 1/4 cup pumpkin seeds
- Salt and pepper to taste

Instructions:

1. Preheat oven to 400°F (200°C).

2. Toss butternut squash with 1 tbsp olive oil, salt, and pepper. Roast for 25-30 minutes.

3. In a bowl, massage kale with remaining olive oil and balsamic vinegar.

4. Add roasted squash and pumpkin seeds. Toss to combine.

Nutrition Information:

- Calories: 180
- Protein: 4g
- Carbohydrates: 25g
- Fat: 10g
- Fiber: 5g
- Sugar: 5g
- Portion Size: 1 cup

Chapter 5: Snacks and Appetizers

Snacking can be both fun and healthy, especially when catering to children with Type 1 Diabetes. This chapter provides a variety of kid-friendly vegetarian snacks and appetizers that are not only delicious but also packed with essential nutrients. These recipes are designed to maintain stable blood sugar levels while ensuring that your child enjoys their food.

Roasted Chickpeas

Ingredients:

- 1 can of chickpeas, drained and rinsed
- 1 tablespoon olive oil
- 1 teaspoon paprika
- 1/2 teaspoon garlic powder
- Salt to taste

Instructions:

1. Preheat the oven to 400°F (200°C).
2. Pat the chickpeas dry with a paper towel.
3. Toss chickpeas with olive oil, paprika, garlic powder, and salt.

4. Spread on a baking sheet and roast for 20-30 minutes, shaking the pan occasionally, until crispy.

Nutrition Information:

- Calories: 180
- Protein: 6g
- Carbohydrates: 24g
- Fat: 6g
- Fiber: 5g
- Sugar: 1g
- Portion size: 1/2 cup

Cucumber and Hummus Bites

Ingredients:

- 1 large cucumber
- 1/2 cup hummus
- 1 tablespoon fresh dill, chopped (optional)

Instructions:

1. Slice the cucumber into thick rounds.
2. Spread a teaspoon of hummus on each cucumber slice.
3. Sprinkle with fresh dill if desired.

Nutrition Information:

- Calories: 50
- Protein: 2g
- Carbohydrates: 6g
- Fat: 2g
- Fiber: 2g
- Sugar: 2g
- Portion size: 6 bites

Apple Slices with Peanut Butter

Ingredients:

- 1 apple, cored and sliced
- 2 tablespoons peanut butter

Instructions:

1. Spread a thin layer of peanut butter on each apple slice.

Nutrition Information:

- Calories: 150
- Protein: 4g
- Carbohydrates: 20g
- Fat: 8g
- Fiber: 4g

- Sugar: 14g
- Portion size: 1 apple

Veggie Sticks with Greek Yogurt Dip

Ingredients:

- 1 cup assorted veggie sticks (carrots, bell peppers, celery)
- 1/2 cup Greek yogurt
- 1 teaspoon lemon juice
- 1/2 teaspoon garlic powder
- Salt and pepper to taste

Instructions:

1. Mix Greek yogurt, lemon juice, garlic powder, salt, and pepper in a small bowl.
2. Serve the dip with veggie sticks.

Nutrition Information:

- Calories: 90
- Protein: 7g
- Carbohydrates: 10g
- Fat: 2g
- Fiber: 3g
- Sugar: 5g

- Portion size: 1 cup veggies with dip

Mini Caprese Skewers

Ingredients:
- 10 cherry tomatoes
- 10 small mozzarella balls
- Fresh basil leaves
- 1 tablespoon balsamic glaze

Instructions:
1. Thread a cherry tomato, mozzarella ball, and basil leaf onto a skewer.
2. Drizzle with balsamic glaze before serving.

Nutrition Information:
- Calories: 120
- Protein: 6g
- Carbohydrates: 4g
- Fat: 8g
- Fiber: 1g
- Sugar: 3g
- Portion size: 5 skewers

Edamame with Sea Salt

Ingredients:

- 1 cup edamame in pods
- 1/2 teaspoon sea salt

Instructions:

1. Steam or boil edamame until tender.
2. Sprinkle with sea salt before serving.

Nutrition Information:

- Calories: 120
- Protein: 11g
- Carbohydrates: 10g
- Fat: 5g
- Fiber: 4g
- Sugar: 2g
- Portion size: 1 cup

Guacamole with Carrot Sticks

Ingredients:

- 2 ripe avocados
- 1 lime, juiced
- 1/4 cup red onion, finely chopped

- 1/4 cup cilantro, chopped
- Salt to taste
- 1 cup carrot sticks

Instructions:

1. Mash avocados in a bowl.
2. Mix in lime juice, red onion, cilantro, and salt.
3. Serve with carrot sticks.

Nutrition Information:

- Calories: 200
- Protein: 2g
- Carbohydrates: 18g
- Fat: 15g
- Fiber: 8g
- Sugar: 5g
- Portion size: 1/4 cup guacamole with carrot sticks

Baked Zucchini Chips

Ingredients:

- 2 zucchinis, thinly sliced
- 1 tablespoon olive oil
- 1/2 teaspoon salt

- 1/2 teaspoon paprika

Instructions:

1. Preheat the oven to 225°F (110°C).

2. Toss zucchini slices with olive oil, salt, and paprika.

3. Arrange on a baking sheet and bake for 1-2 hours until crisp.

Nutrition Information:

- Calories: 50
- Protein: 1g
- Carbohydrates: 5g
- Fat: 3g
- Fiber: 1g
- Sugar: 3g
- Portion size: 1 cup

Almond Flour Crackers with Cheese

Ingredients:

- 1 cup almond flour
- 1 egg
- 1/2 teaspoon salt
- 1/2 teaspoon garlic powder
- 1/4 cup shredded cheese

Instructions:

1. Preheat the oven to 350°F (175°C).

2. Mix almond flour, egg, salt, and garlic powder in a bowl.

3. Roll out the dough between parchment paper.

4. Cut into squares and place on a baking sheet.

5. Bake for 10-12 minutes, then sprinkle cheese on top and bake for another 5 minutes.

Nutrition Information:

- Calories: 150
- Protein: 6g
- Carbohydrates: 4g
- Fat: 12g
- Fiber: 2g
- Sugar: 1g
- Portion size: 5-6 crackers

Stuffed Mini Bell Peppers

Ingredients:

- 10 mini bell peppers
- 1/2 cup cream cheese
- 1/4 cup finely chopped chives
- Salt and pepper to taste

Instructions:

1. Slice the tops off the mini bell peppers and remove seeds.

2. Mix cream cheese with chives, salt, and pepper.

3. Stuff each pepper with the cream cheese mixture.

Nutrition Information:

- Calories: 80

- Protein: 2g

- Carbohydrates: 6g

- Fat: 6g

- Fiber: 1g

- Sugar: 3g

- Portion size: 5 stuffed peppers

Cauliflower Buffalo Bites

Ingredients:

- 1 head cauliflower, cut into florets

- 1/2 cup hot sauce

- 2 tablespoons olive oil

- 1 teaspoon garlic powder

Instructions:

1. Preheat the oven to 400°F (200°C).

2. Toss cauliflower florets with hot sauce, olive oil, and garlic powder.

3. Spread on a baking sheet and bake for 20-25 minutes.

Nutrition Information:

- Calories: 100
- Protein: 3g
- Carbohydrates: 7g
- Fat: 7g
- Fiber: 3g
- Sugar: 2g
- Portion size: 1 cup

Mixed Nuts and Seeds

Ingredients:

- 1/4 cup almonds
- 1/4 cup walnuts
- 1/4 cup pumpkin seeds
- 1/4 cup sunflower seeds

Instructions:

1. Mix all nuts and seeds in a bowl.

Nutrition Information:

- Calories: 200
- Protein: 7g
- Carbohydrates: 8g
- Fat: 18g
- Fiber: 4g
- Sugar: 2g
- Portion size: 1/2 cup

Tofu Nuggets with Dipping Sauce

Ingredients:

- 1 block firm tofu, drained and cubed
- 1/2 cup bread crumbs
- 1/2 teaspoon garlic powder
- 1/2 teaspoon paprika
- Salt and pepper to taste
- 1/4 cup marinara sauce for dipping

Instructions:

1. Preheat the oven to 375°F (190°C).
2. Mix bread crumbs, garlic powder, paprika, salt, and pepper in a bowl.
3. Coat tofu cubes in the mixture and place on a baking sheet.

4. Bake for 20-25 minutes until golden brown.

5. Serve with marinara sauce.

Nutrition Information:

- Calories: 150
- Protein: 8g
- Carbohydrates: 10g
- Fat: 8g
- Fiber: 2g
- Sugar: 2g
- Portion size: 1/2 cup tofu nuggets

Sweet Potato Fries with Cinnamon

Ingredients:

- 2 sweet potatoes, peeled and cut into fries
- 1 tablespoon olive oil
- 1/2 teaspoon cinnamon
- Salt to taste

Instructions:

1. Preheat the oven to 400°F (200°C).

2. Toss sweet potato fries with olive oil, cinnamon, and salt.

3. Spread on a baking sheet and bake for 25-30 minutes until crispy.

Nutrition Information:

- Calories: 150
- Protein: 2g
- Carbohydrates: 30g
- Fat: 4g
- Fiber: 4g
- Sugar: 7g
- Portion size: 1 cup

Fruit Salad with Mint

Ingredients:

- 1 cup strawberries, sliced
- 1 cup blueberries
- 1 cup pineapple chunks
- 1 tablespoon fresh mint, chopped

Instructions:

1. Combine strawberries, blueberries, and pineapple in a bowl.
2. Sprinkle with fresh mint and toss gently.

Nutrition Information:

- Calories: 80
- Protein: 1g
- Carbohydrates: 20g
- Fat: 0.5g
- Fiber: 4g
- Sugar: 16g
- Portion size: 1 cup

Chapter 6: Desserts

Creating delicious and nutritious desserts for kids with Type 1 Diabetes can be a delightful challenge. This chapter offers a collection of desserts that are not only vegetarian and kid-friendly but also mindful of the dietary needs associated with managing diabetes. Each recipe includes nutritional information to help keep track of intake.

Sugar-Free Chocolate Avocado Mousse

Ingredients:

- 2 ripe avocados
- 1/4 cup unsweetened cocoa powder
- 1/4 cup coconut milk
- 2 tablespoons stevia
- 1 teaspoon vanilla extract
- Pinch of salt

Instructions:

1. Blend all ingredients in a food processor until smooth.
2. Chill in the refrigerator for at least 1 hour before serving.

Nutritional Information (per serving):

- Calories: 200
- Protein: 3g
- Carbohydrates: 12g
- Fat: 18g
- Fiber: 7g
- Sugar: 2g
- Portion size: 1/2 cup

Baked Cinnamon Apples

Ingredients:

- 4 medium apples, cored and sliced
- 1 teaspoon ground cinnamon
- 1 tablespoon lemon juice
- 2 tablespoons water

Instructions:

1. Preheat oven to 350°F (175°C).
2. Toss apple slices with cinnamon, lemon juice, and water.
3. Arrange in a baking dish and cover with foil.
4. Bake for 25-30 minutes until tender.

Nutritional Information (per serving):

- Calories: 80
- Protein: 0.5g
- Carbohydrates: 21g
- Fat: 0.3g
- Fiber: 4g
- Sugar: 16g
- Portion size: 1 apple

Chia Seed Pudding with Coconut Milk

Ingredients:

- 1/4 cup chia seeds
- 1 cup coconut milk
- 1 teaspoon vanilla extract
- 1 tablespoon stevia
- Fresh berries for topping

Instructions:

1. Mix chia seeds, coconut milk, vanilla, and stevia in a bowl.
2. Refrigerate for at least 4 hours or overnight.
3. Stir well before serving and top with fresh berries.

Nutritional Information (per serving):

- Calories: 180
- Protein: 3g
- Carbohydrates: 14g
- Fat: 13g
- Fiber: 7g
- Sugar: 2g
- Portion size: 1/2 cup

Greek Yogurt with Honey and Berries

Ingredients:

- 1 cup Greek yogurt
- 1 tablespoon honey
- 1/2 cup mixed berries

Instructions:

1. Spoon yogurt into a bowl.
2. Drizzle with honey.
3. Top with mixed berries.

Nutritional Information (per serving):

- Calories: 150
- Protein: 10g

- Carbohydrates: 22g
- Fat: 4g
- Fiber: 3g
- Sugar: 15g
- Portion size: 1 cup

Almond Flour Brownies

Ingredients:

- 1 cup almond flour
- 1/4 cup unsweetened cocoa powder
- 1/2 cup stevia
- 1/4 teaspoon baking soda
- 1/4 teaspoon salt
- 3 large eggs
- 1/4 cup coconut oil, melted
- 1 teaspoon vanilla extract

Instructions:

1. Preheat oven to 350°F (175°C).
2. Mix almond flour, cocoa powder, stevia, baking soda, and salt.
3. Add eggs, coconut oil, and vanilla extract; stir until combined.

4. Pour into a greased baking pan and bake for 20-25 minutes.

Nutritional Information (per serving):

- Calories: 150
- Protein: 5g
- Carbohydrates: 8g
- Fat: 12g
- Fiber: 3g
- Sugar: 1g
- Portion size: 1 brownie (1/12 of the pan)

Frozen Banana Pops with Dark Chocolate

Ingredients:

- 2 bananas, cut in half
- 1/2 cup dark chocolate chips
- 1 tablespoon coconut oil
- Crushed nuts or coconut flakes (optional)

Instructions:

1. Insert popsicle sticks into banana halves and freeze until solid.
2. Melt dark chocolate chips with coconut oil.

3. Dip frozen bananas in chocolate and sprinkle with nuts or coconut.

4. Freeze until chocolate is set.

Nutritional Information (per serving):

- Calories: 150
- Protein: 1g
- Carbohydrates: 25g
- Fat: 7g
- Fiber: 3g
- Sugar: 15g
- Portion size: 1 banana pop

Carrot and Pineapple Muffins

Ingredients:

- 1 cup grated carrots
- 1/2 cup crushed pineapple, drained
- 1 cup whole wheat flour
- 1/2 cup almond flour
- 1/2 cup stevia
- 1 teaspoon baking soda
- 1/2 teaspoon baking powder
- 1/2 teaspoon cinnamon

- 2 large eggs
- 1/4 cup coconut oil, melted
- 1 teaspoon vanilla extract

Instructions:

1. Preheat oven to 350°F (175°C).
2. Combine dry ingredients in a bowl.
3. Mix wet ingredients in another bowl.
4. Stir wet ingredients into dry until just combined.
5. Fold in carrots and pineapple.
6. Spoon batter into muffin tin and bake for 20-25 minutes.

Nutritional Information (per serving):

- Calories: 140
- Protein: 3g
- Carbohydrates: 18g
- Fat: 6g
- Fiber: 3g
- Sugar: 6g
- Portion size: 1 muffin

Raspberry Sorbet

Ingredients:

- 2 cups fresh raspberries
- 1/4 cup water
- 1/4 cup stevia
- 1 tablespoon lemon juice

Instructions:

1. Blend all ingredients until smooth.
2. Pour into a shallow container and freeze, stirring every 30 minutes until firm.

Nutritional Information (per serving):

- Calories: 70
- Protein: 1g
- Carbohydrates: 18g
- Fat: 0.5g
- Fiber: 6g
- Sugar: 7g
- Portion size: 1/2 cup

Coconut Macaroons

Ingredients:

- 2 cups shredded unsweetened coconut
- 1/4 cup stevia
- 3 egg whites
- 1 teaspoon vanilla extract
- Pinch of salt

Instructions:

1. Preheat oven to 325°F (160°C).
2. Beat egg whites with salt until stiff peaks form.
3. Fold in stevia, coconut, and vanilla.
4. Drop spoonfuls onto a baking sheet and bake for 15-20 minutes.

Nutritional Information (per serving):

- Calories: 60
- Protein: 1g
- Carbohydrates: 3g
- Fat: 5g
- Fiber: 2g
- Sugar: 1g
- Portion size: 1 macaroon

Mango and Lime Sorbet

Ingredients:

- 2 cups frozen mango chunks
- 1/4 cup lime juice
- 1 tablespoon stevia

Instructions:

1. Blend all ingredients until smooth.
2. Serve immediately or freeze until ready to serve.

Nutritional Information (per serving):

- Calories: 80
- Protein: 1g
- Carbohydrates: 21g
- Fat: 0.5g
- Fiber: 2g
- Sugar: 18g
- Portion size: 1/2 cup

Vegan Chocolate Chip Cookies

Ingredients:

- 1 cup almond flour
- 1/2 cup oats

- 1/4 cup stevia
- 1/4 cup coconut oil, melted
- 1 teaspoon vanilla extract
- 1/2 teaspoon baking soda
- 1/4 cup dark chocolate chips

Instructions:

1. Preheat oven to 350°F (175°C).
2. Mix all ingredients in a bowl.
3. Drop spoonfuls onto a baking sheet and flatten slightly.
4. Bake for 10-12 minutes.

Nutritional Information (per serving):

- Calories: 90
- Protein: 2g
- Carbohydrates: 8g
- Fat: 6g
- Fiber: 2g
- Sugar: 2g
- Portion size: 1 cookie

Lemon Blueberry Bars

Ingredients:

- 1 cup almond flour
- 1/4 cup stevia
- 1/4 teaspoon baking soda
- 1/4 teaspoon salt
- 2 large eggs
- 1/4 cup coconut oil, melted
- 1 teaspoon lemon zest
- 1 cup fresh blueberries

Instructions:

1. Preheat oven to 350°F (175°C).
2. Mix almond flour, stevia, baking soda, and salt.
3. Add eggs, coconut oil, and lemon zest; stir until combined.
4. Fold in blueberries and pour into a greased baking pan.
5. Bake for 20-25 minutes.

Nutritional Information (per serving):

- Calories: 120
- Protein: 3g
- Carbohydrates: 9g
- Fat: 9g
- Fiber: 2g

- Sugar: 4g
- Portion size: 1 bar

Strawberry Shortcake

Ingredients:

- 2 cups almond flour
- 1/4 cup stevia
- 1 teaspoon baking powder
- 1/4 teaspoon salt
- 1/4 cup coconut oil, melted
- 2 large eggs
- 1 teaspoon vanilla extract
- 2 cups sliced strawberries
- 1 cup whipped coconut cream

Instructions:

1. Preheat oven to 350°F (175°C).
2. Mix almond flour, stevia, baking powder, and salt.
3. Add coconut oil, eggs, and vanilla; stir until combined.
4. Pour into a greased baking pan and bake for 20-25 minutes.
5. Serve with sliced strawberries and whipped coconut cream.

Nutritional Information (per serving):

- Calories: 180
- Protein: 4g
- Carbohydrates: 12g
- Fat: 14g
- Fiber: 3g
- Sugar: 5g
- Portion size: 1 shortcake

Pomegranate and Orange Salad

Ingredients:

- 1 cup pomegranate seeds
- 2 oranges, peeled and sliced
- 1 tablespoon lemon juice
- 1 tablespoon fresh mint, chopped

Instructions:

1. Combine pomegranate seeds and orange slices in a bowl.
2. Drizzle with lemon juice and sprinkle with fresh mint.
3. Toss gently to combine.

Nutritional Information (per serving):

- Calories: 90

- Protein: 1g
- Carbohydrates: 22g
- Fat: 0.5g
- Fiber: 4g
- Sugar: 18g
- Portion size: 1 cup

Vegan Banana Bread

Ingredients:

- 3 ripe bananas, mashed
- 1/4 cup coconut oil, melted
- 1/4 cup stevia
- 1 teaspoon vanilla extract
- 1 1/2 cups whole wheat flour
- 1 teaspoon baking soda
- 1/4 teaspoon salt
- 1/2 cup chopped walnuts (optional)

Instructions:

1. Preheat oven to 350°F (175°C).
2. Mix mashed bananas, coconut oil, stevia, and vanilla extract.
3. In another bowl, combine whole wheat flour, baking soda, and salt.

4. Stir dry ingredients into wet mixture until just combined.

5. Fold in chopped walnuts, if using.

6. Pour batter into a greased loaf pan and bake for 50-60 minutes.

Nutritional Information (per serving):

- Calories: 150
- Protein: 3g
- Carbohydrates: 22g
- Fat: 7g
- Fiber: 3g
- Sugar: 8g
- Portion size: 1 slice

Chapter 7: Smoothies

Smoothies are a fantastic way to ensure kids with Type 1 Diabetes get the essential nutrients they need. They are easy to prepare, delicious, and packed with vitamins, minerals, and fiber. Here, we provide a collection of kid-friendly, diabetes-friendly vegetarian smoothie recipes that are both nutritious and tasty. Each smoothie is designed to be low in sugar and high in beneficial nutrients, making them perfect for breakfast, a snack, or even a dessert.

Green Detox Smoothie

Ingredients:

- 1 cup spinach
- 1/2 cucumber, sliced
- 1 green apple, chopped
- 1/2 avocado
- 1/2 lemon, juiced
- 1 cup coconut water

Instructions:

1. Combine all ingredients in a blender.
2. Blend until smooth.
3. Serve immediately.

Nutrition Information (per serving):

- Calories: 120
- Protein: 2g
- Carbohydrates: 15g
- Fat: 7g
- Fiber: 5g
- Sugar: 8g
- Portion Size: 1 cup

Berry Blast Smoothie

Ingredients:

- 1/2 cup strawberries
- 1/2 cup blueberries
- 1/2 cup raspberries
- 1/2 banana
- 1 cup almond milk

Instructions:

1. Place all ingredients in a blender.
2. Blend until smooth.
3. Pour into a glass and enjoy.

Nutrition Information (per serving):

- Calories: 140
- Protein: 3g
- Carbohydrates: 28g
- Fat: 3g
- Fiber: 6g
- Sugar: 15g
- Portion Size: 1 cup

Tropical Mango Smoothie

Ingredients:

- 1 cup mango chunks
- 1/2 cup pineapple chunks
- 1/2 banana
- 1 cup coconut milk

Instructions:

1. Blend all ingredients until smooth.
2. Serve chilled.

Nutrition Information (per serving):

- Calories: 180
- Protein: 2g

- Carbohydrates: 32g

- Fat: 7g

- Fiber: 4g

- Sugar: 24g

- Portion Size: 1 cup

Spinach and Pineapple Smoothie

Ingredients:

- 1 cup spinach

- 1 cup pineapple chunks

- 1/2 banana

- 1 cup water

Instructions:

1. Blend spinach, pineapple, banana, and water until smooth.
2. Serve immediately.

Nutrition Information (per serving):

- Calories: 100

- Protein: 1g

- Carbohydrates: 25g

- Fat: 0.5g

- Fiber: 3g

- Sugar: 15g
- Portion Size: 1 cup

Avocado and Lime Smoothie

Ingredients:

- 1/2 avocado
- 1/2 banana
- 1 cup spinach
- 1/2 lime, juiced
- 1 cup water

Instructions:

1. Blend avocado, banana, spinach, lime juice, and water until smooth.
2. Serve immediately.

Nutrition Information (per serving):

- Calories: 150
- Protein: 2g
- Carbohydrates: 19g
- Fat: 8g
- Fiber: 6g
- Sugar: 8g

- Portion Size: 1 cup

Strawberry Banana Smoothie

Ingredients:

- 1/2 cup strawberries
- 1/2 banana
- 1/2 cup Greek yogurt
- 1/2 cup almond milk

Instructions:

1. Blend strawberries, banana, Greek yogurt, and almond milk until smooth.
2. Serve chilled.

Nutrition Information (per serving):

- Calories: 130
- Protein: 6g
- Carbohydrates: 22g
- Fat: 2g
- Fiber: 3g
- Sugar: 14g
- Portion Size: 1 cup

Blueberry Almond Smoothie

Ingredients:

- 1/2 cup blueberries
- 1 tablespoon almond butter
- 1/2 banana
- 1 cup almond milk

Instructions:

1. Blend blueberries, almond butter, banana, and almond milk until smooth.
2. Serve immediately.

Nutrition Information (per serving):

- Calories: 180
- Protein: 4g
- Carbohydrates: 22g
- Fat: 8g
- Fiber: 4g
- Sugar: 14g
- Portion Size: 1 cup

Chocolate Peanut Butter Smoothie

Ingredients:

- 1 tablespoon unsweetened cocoa powder
- 1 tablespoon peanut butter
- 1/2 banana
- 1 cup unsweetened almond milk

Instructions:

1. Blend cocoa powder, peanut butter, banana, and almond milk until smooth.
2. Serve chilled.

Nutrition Information (per serving):

- Calories: 200
- Protein: 5g
- Carbohydrates: 24g
- Fat: 10g
- Fiber: 4g
- Sugar: 12g
- Portion Size: 1 cup

Kale and Apple Smoothie

Ingredients:

- 1 cup kale
- 1/2 apple, chopped
- 1/2 banana
- 1 cup water

Instructions:

1. Blend kale, apple, banana, and water until smooth.
2. Serve immediately.

Nutrition Information (per serving):

- Calories: 90
- Protein: 1g
- Carbohydrates: 22g
- Fat: 0.5g
- Fiber: 3g
- Sugar: 14g
- Portion Size: 1 cup

Peach and Oat Smoothie

Ingredients:

- 1/2 cup peaches, chopped

- 1/4 cup rolled oats
- 1/2 banana
- 1 cup almond milk

Instructions:

1. Blend peaches, rolled oats, banana, and almond milk until smooth.
2. Serve immediately.

Nutrition Information (per serving):

- Calories: 150
- Protein: 3g
- Carbohydrates: 30g
- Fat: 3g
- Fiber: 4g
- Sugar: 14g
- Portion Size: 1 cup

Watermelon Mint Smoothie

Ingredients:

- 1 cup watermelon chunks
- 1/2 cup cucumber, sliced
- 1 tablespoon fresh mint leaves

- 1 cup water

Instructions:

1. Blend watermelon, cucumber, mint leaves, and water until smooth.
2. Serve chilled.

Nutrition Information (per serving):

- Calories: 60
- Protein: 1g
- Carbohydrates: 15g
- Fat: 0g
- Fiber: 1g
- Sugar: 11g
- Portion Size: 1 cup

Carrot Ginger Smoothie

Ingredients:

- 1/2 cup carrots, chopped
- 1/2 banana
- 1/2 teaspoon grated ginger
- 1 cup orange juice

Instructions:

1. Blend carrots, banana, ginger, and orange juice until smooth.

2. Serve immediately.

Nutrition Information (per serving):

- Calories: 110

- Protein: 1g

- Carbohydrates: 27g

- Fat: 0.5g

- Fiber: 3g

- Sugar: 18g

- Portion Size: 1 cup

Coconut Pineapple Smoothie

Ingredients:

- 1 cup pineapple chunks

- 1/2 cup coconut milk

- 1/2 banana

- 1/2 teaspoon vanilla extract

Instructions:

1. Blend pineapple, coconut milk, banana, and vanilla extract until smooth.

2. Serve chilled.

Nutrition Information (per serving):

- Calories: 160
- Protein: 1g
- Carbohydrates: 28g
- Fat: 6g
- Fiber: 3g
- Sugar: 18g
- Portion Size: 1 cup

Pumpkin Pie Smoothie

Ingredients:

- 1/2 cup pumpkin puree
- 1/2 banana
- 1/2 teaspoon pumpkin pie spice
- 1 cup unsweetened almond milk

Instructions:

1. Blend pumpkin puree, banana, pumpkin pie spice, and almond milk until smooth.
2. Serve immediately.

Nutrition Information (per serving):

- Calories: 90
- Protein: 2g
- Carbohydrates: 18g
- Fat: 2g
- Fiber: 3g
- Sugar: 9g
- Portion Size: 1 cup

Cherry Vanilla Smoothie

Ingredients:

- 1/2 cup cherries, pitted
- 1/2 banana
- 1/2 teaspoon vanilla extract
- 1 cup almond milk

Instructions:

1. Blend cherries, banana, vanilla extract, and almond milk until smooth.
2. Serve chilled.

Nutrition Information (per serving):

- Calories: 120

- Protein: 2g
- Carbohydrates: 26g
- Fat: 2g
- Fiber: 3g
- Sugar: 18g
- Portion Size: 1 cup

CONCLUSION

Thank you for exploring our collection of Type 1 Diabetes Kid-Friendly Vegetarian Recipes. This book was crafted with care to empower families navigating the journey of managing diabetes in children while embracing the benefits of a vegetarian lifestyle. Throughout these pages, we've shared nutritious and delicious recipes that prioritize balance, flavor, and simplicity.

By focusing on whole foods and mindful eating, these recipes aim to support stable blood sugar levels and promote overall well-being. We understand the challenges of ensuring variety and nutrition in everyday meals, especially when dietary restrictions are involved. That's why each recipe in this book is not only kid-friendly but also designed to be easily integrated into daily life.

As you embark on this culinary journey, remember that small changes can make a big difference. Whether you're preparing a hearty breakfast, a satisfying lunch, or a tempting dessert, each meal presents an opportunity to nourish and delight. By choosing wholesome ingredients and thoughtful preparation methods, you're providing your child with the foundation for a healthy future.

We hope these recipes inspire creativity in your kitchen and foster moments of joy around the dining table. Remember, managing diabetes is a journey, and you're not alone. With dedication, support, and delicious food, we can empower our children to thrive, one meal at a time.

Here's to health, happiness, and the shared love of good food!